LOW OXALATE COOKBOOK

Healthy, Kidney-Friendly Recipes for Every Occasion

Dr Lily Morgan

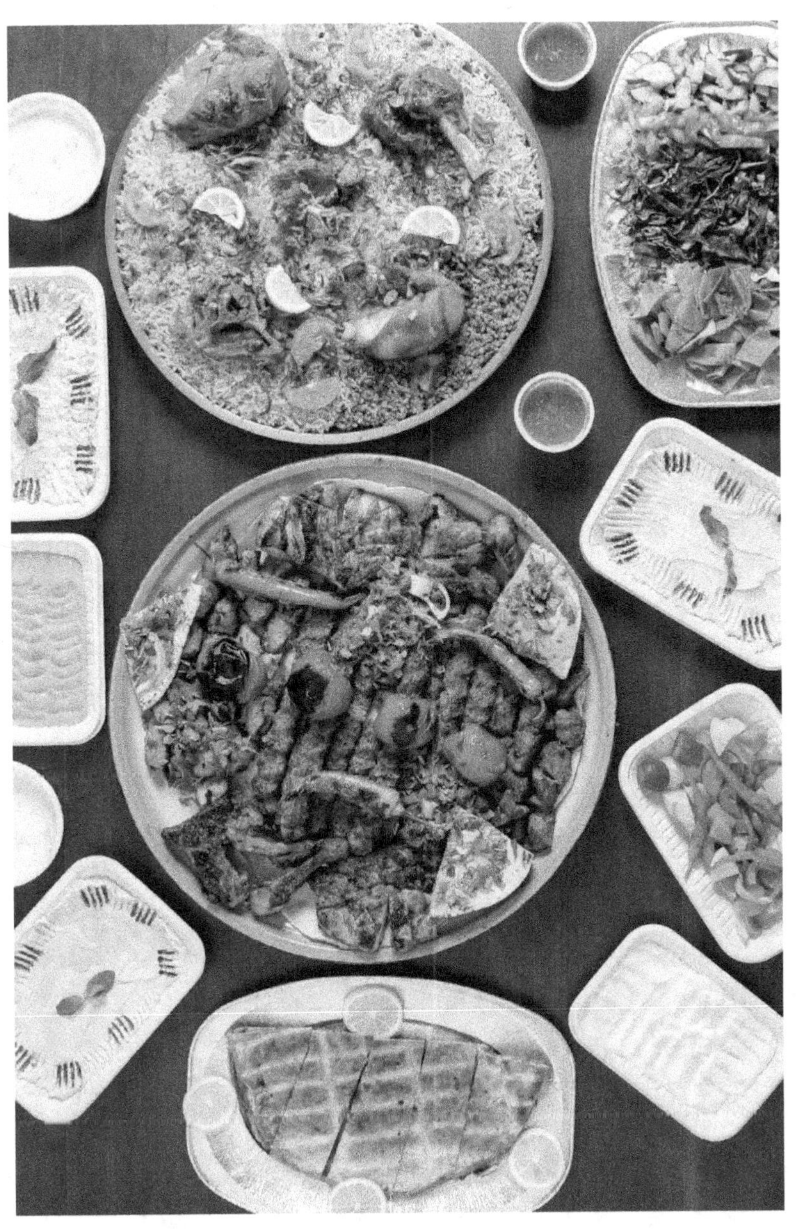

TABLE OF CONTENTS

INTRODUCTION 9

Benefits of a Low Oxalate Diet 10

Chapter 1: 30 Day Meal Plan 13

Week 1: 13

Week 2 15

Week 3 17

Week 4 20

Chapter 2: Breakfast Recipes........................24

Low Oxalate Smoothie Bowl................................ 24

Scrambled Eggs with Spinach 25

Banana Oat Pancakes 26

Greek Yogurt Parfait.. 27

Avocado and Tomato Breakfast Wrap.................. 27

Almond Butter Oatmeal...................................... 28

Veggie Omelette 29

Blueberry Breakfast Quinoa 30

Chia Seed Pudding... 31

Spinach and Feta Quiche 32

Breakfast Tacos... 33

Apple Cinnamon Oat Bran.................................. 33

Coconut Milk Rice Pudding................................. 34

Zucchini and Mushroom Frittata 35

Sweet Potato Hash 36

Cottage Cheese and Fruit Bowl 37

Buckwheat Pancakes 38

Broccoli and Cheese Breakfast Casserole.................... 39

Chapter 3: Lunch Recipes.......................................41

Turkey and Avocado Wrap.............................. 41

Spinach and Strawberry Salad 42

Quinoa and Black Bean Salad........................ 42

Tuna Salad Lettuce Wraps 43

Chickpea and Vegetable Stir-Fry...................... 44

Caprese Salad.. 45

Lentil and Vegetable Soup.............................. 46

Chicken and Vegetable Bowl........................... 47

Egg Salad Lettuce Wraps................................ 48

Cauliflower Rice Stir-Fry 49

Greek Salad.. 50

Zucchini Noodles with Pesto 51

Turkey and Vegetable Soup............................ 52

Cucumber and Tomato Salad.......................... 53

Shrimp and Avocado Salad............................. 54

Broccoli and Cheddar Stuffed Chicken 55

Spinach and Mushroom Quiche....................... 56

Quinoa and Vegetable Bowl 57

Chapter 4: Dinner Recipes 59

Grilled Lemon Herb Chicken.......................... 59

Baked Salmon with Dill.......................... 60

Stir-Fried Tofu with Broccoli 61

Lemon Garlic Shrimp 62

Roasted Vegetable Medley 63

Turkey Meatballs in Tomato Sauce 64

Baked Cod with Herbs 65

Beef and Broccoli Stir-Fry.......................... 66

Spaghetti Squash with Pesto 67

Pork Tenderloin with Apple Glaze 68

Baked Eggplant Parmesan 69

Chicken and Asparagus Stir-Fry.......................... 70

Grilled Portobello Mushrooms 71

Stuffed Bell Peppers 72

Balsamic Glazed Brussels Sprouts.......................... 73

Cilantro Lime Cauliflower Rice.......................... 74

Lemon Butter Tilapia.......................... 75

Ratatouille.......................... 76

Chapter 5: Snacks and Appetizers 78

Guacamole with Veggie Sticks.......................... 78

Hummus and Carrot Slices 79

Greek Yogurt with Berries.......................... 80

Cucumber Slices with Tzatziki 81

Almonds and Dried Cranberries 82

Roasted Red Pepper Dip 82

Deviled Eggs 83

Cottage Cheese with Pineapple.................................. 84

Stuffed Mushrooms.. 85

Edamame with Sea Salt 86

Avocado Salsa.. 86

Baked Sweet Potato Fries 87

Caprese Skewers 88

Mixed Nuts... 89

Cucumber and Cream Cheese Roll-Ups 89

Sliced Bell Peppers with Ranch Dressing.................... 90

Zucchini Chips 91

Kale Chips.. 91

Chapter 6: Desserts 93

Low Oxalate Berry Sorbet 93

Chocolate Avocado Mousse 94

Almond Flour Brownies 94

Baked Apple with Cinnamon.. 95

Lemon Poppy Seed Cake 96

Coconut Milk Ice Cream.. 97

Banana Nut Muffins.. 98

Greek Yogurt with Honey and Nuts 99

Chia Seed Chocolate Pudding...................................... 99

Strawberry Shortcake 100

Pumpkin Pie Bites 101

Mango Sorbet 102

Raspberry Cheesecake Bars 103

Almond and Date Energy Balls 104

Carrot Cake Bites 104

Blueberry Crumble 105

Chocolate-Dipped Strawberries 106

Pecan Pie Squares 107

CONCLUSION 108

Your Journey, Your Success 108

Staying on a Low Oxalate Diet 108

Tips for Long-Term Success 109

INTRODUCTION

Oxalates are naturally occurring compounds found in a wide range of foods we consume daily. These organic acids serve various biological functions in plants, but when they accumulate excessively in our bodies, they can lead to health issues. Understanding the role of oxalates and their impact on our well-being is crucial for making informed dietary choices.

Oxalates in our diet primarily come from foods like spinach, rhubarb, beets, nuts, and certain grains. They are often present in foods touted for their health benefits, which can make navigating a low oxalate diet seem daunting. However, the potential impact of oxalates on our health cannot be ignored.

One significant concern is the formation of oxalate crystals. In some individuals, especially those prone to kidney stones, high levels of oxalates in the body can lead to the crystallization of calcium oxalate, a substance known for its role in kidney stone formation. These crystals can accumulate in the urinary tract, causing painful stones that may require medical intervention.

Moreover, oxalates can interfere with the absorption of essential minerals like calcium and magnesium in the digestive system. This can have a cascading effect on bone health and overall nutrient balance. Over time, an excess of oxalates can contribute to the development of conditions such as osteoporosis.

Benefits of a Low Oxalate Diet

Embarking on a low oxalate diet can offer a range of potential benefits, particularly for those at risk of oxalate-related health issues:

1. **Reduced Risk of Kidney Stones**: By limiting dietary oxalates, individuals with a history of kidney stones can significantly lower their risk of stone formation. This can translate to less pain, fewer medical procedures, and an improved quality of life.

2. **Better Mineral Absorption:** A low oxalate diet can enhance the body's ability to absorb essential

minerals like calcium and magnesium. This is vital for maintaining strong bones and overall mineral balance.

3. **Improved Gut Health**: Some people may experience digestive discomfort or issues related to high oxalate intake. A low oxalate diet can alleviate these problems, promoting better gut health and comfort.

4. **Potential Pain Reduction**: For individuals with conditions like vulvodynia or interstitial cystitis, reducing dietary oxalates may lead to a decrease in pain and discomfort associated with these conditions.

5. **Customized Nutritional Approach**: A low oxalate diet encourages a shift towards foods that are naturally lower in oxalates. This often means increased consumption of fruits, vegetables, and grains that are gentle on the digestive system and supportive of overall health.

It's important to note that adopting a low oxalate diet should be done under the guidance of a healthcare professional, especially if you have specific medical conditions.

Balancing nutritional needs while reducing oxalate intake requires careful planning and consideration.

In summary, understanding oxalates and their impact on our health is a fundamental step toward making informed dietary choices. While oxalates are present in many foods, a low oxalate diet can be a valuable tool for managing specific health conditions and promoting overall well-being. It's a personalized approach to nutrition that empowers individuals to take control of their health and live more comfortably.

Chapter 1: 30 Day Meal Plan

Week 1:

Day 1:

- Breakfast: Low Oxalate Smoothie Bowl
- Lunch: Turkey and Avocado Wrap
- Dinner: Grilled Lemon Herb Chicken
- Snacks: Guacamole with Veggie Sticks
- Dessert: Low Oxalate Berry Sorbet

Day 2:

- Breakfast: Scrambled Eggs with Spinach
- Lunch: Spinach and Strawberry Salad
- Dinner: Baked Salmon with Dill
- Snacks: Hummus and Carrot Slices
- Dessert: Chocolate Avocado Mousse

Day 3:

- Breakfast: Banana Oat Pancakes
- Lunch: Quinoa and Black Bean Salad
- Dinner: Stir-Fried Tofu with Broccoli

- Snacks: Greek Yogurt with Berries
- Dessert: Almond Flour Brownies

Day 4:

- Breakfast: Greek Yogurt Parfait
- Lunch: Tuna Salad Lettuce Wraps
- Dinner: Lemon Garlic Shrimp
- Snacks: Cucumber Slices with Tzatziki
- Dessert: Baked Apple with Cinnamon

Day 5:

- Breakfast: Avocado and Tomato Breakfast Wrap
- Lunch: Chickpea and Vegetable Stir-Fry
- Dinner: Roasted Vegetable Medley
- Snacks: Almonds and Dried Cranberries
- Dessert: Lemon Poppy Seed Cake

Day 6:

- Breakfast: Almond Butter Oatmeal
- Lunch: Caprese Salad
- Dinner: Turkey Meatballs in Tomato Sauce
- Snacks: Roasted Red Pepper Dip

- Dessert: Coconut Milk Ice Cream

Day 7:

- Breakfast: Veggie Omelette
- Lunch: Lentil and Vegetable Soup
- Dinner: Baked Cod with Herbs
- Snacks: Deviled Eggs
- Dessert: Banana Nut Muffins

Week 2

Day 8:

- Breakfast: Blueberry Breakfast Quinoa
- Lunch: Chicken and Vegetable Bowl
- Dinner: Beef and Broccoli Stir-Fry
- Snacks: Cottage Cheese with Pineapple
- Dessert: Greek Yogurt with Honey and Nuts

Day 9:

- Breakfast: Chia Seed Pudding
- Lunch: Egg Salad Lettuce Wraps
- Dinner: Spaghetti Squash with Pesto
- Snacks: Stuffed Mushrooms

- Dessert: Chia Seed Chocolate Pudding

Day 10:

- Breakfast: Spinach and Feta Quiche
- Lunch: Cauliflower Rice Stir-Fry
- Dinner: Pork Tenderloin with Apple Glaze
- Snacks: Edamame with Sea Salt
- Dessert: Strawberry Shortcake

Day 11:

- Breakfast: Breakfast Tacos
- Lunch: Greek Salad
- Dinner: Baked Eggplant Parmesan
- Snacks: Avocado Salsa
- Dessert: Pumpkin Pie Bites

Day 12:

- Breakfast: Apple Cinnamon Oat Bran
- Lunch: Zucchini Noodles with Pesto
- Dinner: Chicken and Asparagus Stir-Fry
- Snacks: Baked Sweet Potato Fries
- Dessert: Mango Sorbet

Day 13:

- Breakfast: Coconut Milk Rice Pudding
- Lunch: Turkey and Vegetable Soup
- Dinner: Grilled Portobello Mushrooms
- Snacks: Caprese Skewers
- Dessert: Raspberry Cheesecake Bars

Day 14:

- Breakfast: Zucchini and Mushroom Frittata
- Lunch: Cucumber and Tomato Salad
- Dinner: Stuffed Bell Peppers
- Snacks: Mixed Nuts
- Dessert: Almond and Date Energy Balls

Week 3

Day 15:

- Breakfast: Carrot Cake Bites
- Lunch: Shrimp and Avocado Salad
- Dinner: Balsamic Glazed Brussels Sprouts
- Snacks: Cucumber and Cream Cheese Roll-Ups
- Dessert: Blueberry Crumble

Day 16:

- Breakfast: Sweet Potato Hash
- Lunch: Broccoli and Cheddar Stuffed Chicken
- Dinner: Cilantro Lime Cauliflower Rice
- Snacks: Sliced Bell Peppers with Ranch Dressing
- Dessert: Chocolate-Dipped Strawberries

Day 17:

- Breakfast: Cottage Cheese and Fruit Bowl
- Lunch: Spinach and Mushroom Quiche
- Dinner: Lemon Butter Tilapia
- Snacks: Zucchini Chips
- Dessert: Pecan Pie Squares

Day 18:

- Breakfast: Buckwheat Pancakes
- Lunch: Quinoa and Vegetable Bowl
- Dinner: Ratatouille
- Snacks: Kale Chips
- Dessert: Low Oxalate Berry Sorbet

Day 19:

- Breakfast: Low Oxalate Smoothie Bowl
- Lunch: Turkey and Avocado Wrap
- Dinner: Grilled Lemon Herb Chicken
- Snacks: Guacamole with Veggie Sticks
- Dessert: Chocolate Avocado Mousse

Day 20:

- Breakfast: Scrambled Eggs with Spinach
- Lunch: Spinach and Strawberry Salad
- Dinner: Baked Salmon with Dill
- Snacks: Hummus and Carrot Slices
- Dessert: Almond Flour Brownies

Day 21:

- Breakfast: Banana Oat Pancakes
- Lunch: Quinoa and Black Bean Salad
- Dinner: Stir-Fried Tofu with Broccoli
- Snacks: Greek Yogurt with Berries
- Dessert: Baked Apple with Cinnamon

Week 4

Day 22:

- Breakfast: Greek Yogurt Parfait
- Lunch: Tuna Salad Lettuce Wraps
- Dinner: Lemon Garlic Shrimp
- Snacks: Cucumber Slices with Tzatziki
- Dessert: Baked Apple with Cinnamon

Day 23:

- Breakfast: Avocado and Tomato Breakfast Wrap
- Lunch: Chickpea and Vegetable Stir-Fry
- Dinner: Roasted Vegetable Medley
- Snacks: Almonds and Dried Cranberries
- Dessert: Lemon Poppy Seed Cake

Day 24:

- Breakfast: Almond Butter Oatmeal
- Lunch: Caprese Salad
- Dinner: Turkey Meatballs in Tomato Sauce
- Snacks: Roasted Red Pepper Dip
- Dessert: Coconut Milk Ice Cream

Day 25:

- Breakfast: Veggie Omelette
- Lunch: Lentil and Vegetable Soup
- Dinner: Baked Cod with Herbs
- Snacks: Deviled Eggs
- Dessert: Banana Nut Muffins

Day 26:

- Breakfast: Blueberry Breakfast Quinoa
- Lunch: Chicken and Vegetable Bowl
- Dinner: Beef and Broccoli Stir-Fry
- Snacks: Cottage Cheese with Pineapple
- Dessert: Greek Yogurt with Honey and Nuts

Day 27:

- Breakfast: Chia Seed Pudding
- Lunch: Egg Salad Lettuce Wraps
- Dinner: Spaghetti Squash with Pesto
- Snacks: Stuffed Mushrooms
- Dessert: Chia Seed Chocolate Pudding

Day 28:

- Breakfast: Spinach and Feta Quiche
- Lunch: Cauliflower Rice Stir-Fry
- Dinner: Pork Tenderloin with Apple Glaze
- Snacks: Edamame with Sea Salt
- Dessert: Strawberry Shortcake

Day 29:

- Breakfast: Breakfast Tacos
- Lunch: Greek Salad
- Dinner: Baked Eggplant Parmesan
- Snacks: Avocado Salsa
- Dessert: Pumpkin Pie Bites

Day 30:

- Breakfast: Apple Cinnamon Oat Bran
- Lunch: Zucchini Noodles with Pesto
- Dinner: Chicken and Asparagus Stir-Fry
- Snacks: Baked Sweet Potato Fries
- Dessert: Mango Sorbet

Congratulations on completing your 30-day low oxalate meal plan! This plan offers a wide variety of delicious and nutritious options to help you maintain a low oxalate diet. Enjoy your meals and the benefits of this dietary choice.

Chapter 2: Breakfast Recipes

These morning delights are not only nutritious but also brimming with flavor. From hearty omelettes to sweet and satisfying oatmeal, there's something here to please every palate. So, rise and shine as we explore these nourishing low oxalate breakfast options.

Low Oxalate Smoothie Bowl

Ingredients:

- 1/2 cup spinach
- 1/2 banana
- 1/2 cup blueberries
- 1/2 cup Greek yogurt
- 1/4 cup almond milk
- 1 tablespoon almond butter
- 1 teaspoon honey (optional)
- Sliced almonds and fresh berries for topping

Instructions:

1. In a blender, combine spinach, banana, blueberries, Greek yogurt, almond milk, almond butter, and honey (if desired).

2. Blend until smooth.

3. Pour into a bowl and top with sliced almonds and fresh berries.

Scrambled Eggs with Spinach

Ingredients:

- 2 eggs
- 1/4 cup fresh spinach, chopped
- Salt and pepper to taste
- 1 teaspoon olive oil

Instructions:

1. Heat olive oil in a non-stick skillet over medium heat.

2. Whisk eggs in a bowl and add chopped spinach, salt, and pepper.

3. Pour the egg mixture into the skillet and cook, stirring gently, until eggs are scrambled and spinach is wilted.

Banana Oat Pancakes

Ingredients:

- 1 ripe banana, mashed
- 1/2 cup oats
- 1/4 cup almond milk
- 1/2 teaspoon cinnamon
- 1/2 teaspoon vanilla extract
- 1 egg (optional)
- Cooking spray or oil for the pan

Instructions:

1. In a bowl, combine mashed banana, oats, almond milk, cinnamon, and vanilla extract. If desired, add an egg for extra fluffiness.
2. Heat a skillet over medium heat and lightly grease with cooking spray or oil.
3. Pour pancake batter onto the skillet to form small pancakes.
4. Cook until bubbles form on the surface, then flip and cook until golden brown.

Greek Yogurt Parfait

Ingredients:

- 1/2 cup Greek yogurt
- 1/4 cup low oxalate berries (e.g., strawberries, blueberries)
- 1 tablespoon honey
- 2 tablespoons granola

Instructions:

1. In a glass or bowl, layer Greek yogurt, berries, honey, and granola.
2. Repeat the layers as desired.
3. Enjoy this delicious and healthy parfait!

Avocado and Tomato Breakfast Wrap

Ingredients:

- 1 whole-grain tortilla
- 1 ripe avocado, sliced
- 1 ripe tomato, sliced
- 2 eggs, scrambled

- Salt and pepper to taste
- Salsa (optional)

Instructions:

1. Warm the tortilla in a dry skillet or microwave for a few seconds.
2. In a separate skillet, scramble the eggs until they are cooked to your liking.
3. Lay the warm tortilla flat and add slices of avocado, tomato, and scrambled eggs.
4. Season with salt and pepper.
5. If you like a little extra kick, add salsa.
6. Roll up the tortilla and enjoy your nutritious breakfast wrap.

Almond Butter Oatmeal

Ingredients:

- 1/2 cup oats
- 1 cup almond milk
- 1 tablespoon almond butter
- 1 teaspoon honey (optional)
- Sliced almonds for topping

Instructions:

1. Combine oats and almond milk in a saucepan.

2. Cook over medium heat, stirring occasionally, until the oatmeal reaches your desired consistency.

3. Stir in almond butter and honey (if desired).

4. Serve hot, topped with sliced almonds.

Veggie Omelette

Ingredients:

- 2 eggs
- 1/4 cup diced bell peppers
- 1/4 cup diced tomatoes
- 1/4 cup diced onions
- 1/4 cup shredded low oxalate cheese (e.g., cheddar)
- Salt and pepper to taste
- Cooking spray or oil for the pan

Instructions:

1. Heat a non-stick skillet over medium-high heat and grease with cooking spray or oil.

2. In a bowl, whisk eggs and season with salt and pepper.

3. Pour the whisked eggs into the skillet.

4. As the eggs start to set, add the diced vegetables and shredded cheese on one half of the omelette.

5. Fold the other half over the filling and cook until the cheese is melted and the omelette is cooked through.

Blueberry Breakfast Quinoa

Ingredients:

- 1/2 cup quinoa
- 1 cup water
- 1/2 cup fresh blueberries
- 1 tablespoon honey (optional)
- 1/4 cup chopped nuts (e.g., almonds, walnuts)

Instructions:

1. Rinse the quinoa under cold water.

2. In a saucepan, combine quinoa and water and bring to a boil.

3. Reduce heat to low, cover, and simmer for about 15 minutes or until quinoa is cooked and water is absorbed.

4. Remove from heat and fluff with a fork.

5. Top with fresh blueberries, drizzle with honey (if desired), and sprinkle with chopped nuts.

Chia Seed Pudding

Ingredients:

- 2 tablespoons chia seeds
- 1/2 cup almond milk
- 1/2 teaspoon vanilla extract
- 1 tablespoon honey (optional)
- Fresh berries for topping

Instructions:

1. In a bowl, mix chia seeds, almond milk, vanilla extract, and honey (if desired).
2. Stir well and refrigerate for at least 2 hours or overnight.
3. Before serving, top with fresh berries for a burst of flavor.

Spinach and Feta Quiche

Ingredients:

- 1 pre-made pie crust (store-bought or homemade)
- 1 cup fresh spinach, chopped
- 1/2 cup crumbled feta cheese
- 4 eggs
- 1 cup milk
- Salt and pepper to taste

Instructions:

1. Preheat your oven to 375°F (190°C).
2. Place the pie crust in a pie dish.
3. Sprinkle chopped spinach and crumbled feta evenly over the crust.
4. In a bowl, whisk together eggs, milk, salt, and pepper.
5. Pour the egg mixture over the spinach and feta.
6. Bake in the preheated oven for about 30-35 minutes, or until the quiche is set and the top is golden brown.

Breakfast Tacos

Ingredients:

- 2 small whole-grain tortillas
- 2 eggs, scrambled
- 1/4 cup diced tomatoes
- 1/4 cup diced bell peppers
- 2 tablespoons chopped cilantro
- Salsa (optional)
- Avocado slices (optional)

Instructions:

1. Warm the tortillas in a dry skillet or microwave for a few seconds.
2. Fill each tortilla with scrambled eggs, diced tomatoes, diced bell peppers, and chopped cilantro.
3. If desired, add a dollop of salsa and avocado slices.
4. Fold the tortillas and enjoy your breakfast tacos.

Apple Cinnamon Oat Bran

Ingredients:

- 1/2 cup oat bran

- 1 cup water
- 1/2 apple, diced
- 1/2 teaspoon ground cinnamon
- 1 tablespoon honey (optional)

Instructions:

1. In a saucepan, combine oat bran and water.
2. Bring to a boil, then reduce heat and simmer for about 5 minutes or until oat bran is cooked and thickened.
3. Stir in diced apple, ground cinnamon, and honey (if desired).
4. Cook for an additional 2-3 minutes until the apple is tender.
5. Serve warm and enjoy the comforting flavors.

Coconut Milk Rice Pudding

Ingredients:

- 1/2 cup Arborio rice
- 1 1/2 cups coconut milk
- 1/4 cup sugar (or sweetener of your choice)
- 1/2 teaspoon vanilla extract

- Shredded coconut and sliced almonds for topping

Instructions:

1. In a saucepan, combine Arborio rice and coconut milk.
2. Cook over medium heat, stirring occasionally, until the rice is tender and the mixture thickens (about 25-30 minutes).
3. Stir in sugar (or sweetener) and vanilla extract.
4. Remove from heat and let it cool slightly.
5. Serve warm or chilled, topped with shredded coconut and sliced almonds.

Zucchini and Mushroom Frittata

Ingredients:

- 4 eggs
- 1/2 cup diced zucchini
- 1/2 cup sliced mushrooms
- 1/4 cup diced onions
- 1/4 cup shredded low oxalate cheese (e.g., mozzarella)
- Salt and pepper to taste

- Cooking spray or oil for the pan

Instructions:

1. Preheat your oven to 350°F (175°C).
2. In a bowl, whisk eggs and season with salt and pepper.
3. Heat an oven-safe skillet over medium heat and grease with cooking spray or oil.
4. Add diced zucchini, sliced mushrooms, and diced onions to the skillet. Sauté until tender.
5. Pour the whisked eggs over the vegetables and sprinkle with shredded cheese.
6. Transfer the skillet to the preheated oven and bake for about 15-20 minutes, or until the frittata is set and golden brown on top.

Sweet Potato Hash

Ingredients:

- 1 sweet potato, peeled and diced
- 1/2 cup diced bell peppers
- 1/4 cup diced onions
- 1/4 teaspoon paprika

- Salt and pepper to taste
- Cooking oil for the pan

Instructions:

1. Heat a skillet over medium heat and add cooking oil.
2. Add diced sweet potato, bell peppers, and onions to the skillet.
3. Season with paprika, salt, and pepper.
4. Sauté until the sweet potato is cooked through and slightly crispy.

Cottage Cheese and Fruit Bowl

Ingredients:

- 1/2 cup low-fat cottage cheese
- 1/2 cup diced low oxalate fruits (e.g., strawberries, kiwi)
- 1 tablespoon honey (optional)
- Chopped nuts (e.g., almonds, walnuts) for topping

Instructions:

1. In a bowl, combine low-fat cottage cheese and diced fruits.

2. Drizzle with honey (if desired) and top with chopped nuts for added crunch and flavor.

Buckwheat Pancakes

Ingredients:

- 1/2 cup buckwheat flour
- 1/2 teaspoon baking powder
- 1 egg
- 1/2 cup almond milk
- 1 tablespoon honey (optional)
- Sliced bananas for topping

Instructions:

1. In a bowl, mix buckwheat flour and baking powder.
2. In another bowl, whisk egg, almond milk, and honey (if desired).
3. Combine wet and dry ingredients and stir until well mixed.
4. Heat a skillet over medium heat and lightly grease with cooking spray or oil.

5. Pour pancake batter onto the skillet and cook until bubbles form on the surface, then flip and cook until golden brown.

6. Top with sliced bananas for a naturally sweet twist.

Broccoli and Cheese Breakfast Casserole

Ingredients:

- 2 cups chopped broccoli
- 1/2 cup shredded low oxalate cheese (e.g., cheddar)
- 6 eggs
- 1/2 cup milk
- Salt and pepper to taste

Instructions:

1. Preheat your oven to 350°F (175°C).
2. Steam the chopped broccoli until slightly tender.
3. In a baking dish, spread out the steamed broccoli and sprinkle with shredded cheese.
4. In a bowl, whisk eggs, milk, salt, and pepper.
5. Pour the egg mixture over the broccoli and cheese.

6. Bake in the preheated oven for about 25-30 minutes, or until the casserole is set and the top is golden brown.

Chapter 3: Lunch Recipes

In this chapter, we explore a delightful array of lunch recipes designed to tickle your taste buds while adhering to a low oxalate diet. These dishes combine fresh ingredients and creative flavors to ensure that your midday meal is both satisfying and nutritious.

Turkey and Avocado Wrap

Ingredients:

- 1 large whole-wheat tortilla
- 3 ounces of sliced turkey breast
- 1/2 avocado, sliced
- 1/4 cup baby spinach leaves
- 1 tablespoon Greek yogurt
- 1 teaspoon Dijon mustard
- Salt and pepper to taste

Instructions:

1. Lay out the tortilla and spread Greek yogurt and Dijon mustard evenly over it.

2. Place turkey slices, avocado, and spinach on top.

3. Season with salt and pepper.

4. Roll up the tortilla tightly, slice in half, and enjoy.

Spinach and Strawberry Salad

Ingredients:

- 2 cups fresh baby spinach
- 1 cup sliced strawberries
- 1/4 cup sliced almonds
- 2 tablespoons balsamic vinaigrette dressing

Instructions:

1. In a bowl, combine spinach, sliced strawberries, and sliced almonds.

2. Drizzle with balsamic vinaigrette dressing.

3. Toss gently to coat, and your refreshing salad is ready to serve.

Quinoa and Black Bean Salad

Ingredients:

- 1 cup cooked quinoa, cooled

- 1 cup canned black beans, drained and rinsed
- 1/2 cup diced red bell pepper
- 1/4 cup chopped fresh cilantro
- 2 tablespoons lime juice
- 1 tablespoon olive oil
- Salt and pepper to taste

Instructions:

1. In a large bowl, combine quinoa, black beans, red bell pepper, and cilantro.
2. In a separate small bowl, whisk together lime juice, olive oil, salt, and pepper.
3. Pour the dressing over the salad and toss to mix well. Serve chilled.

Tuna Salad Lettuce Wraps

Ingredients:

- 1 can (5 ounces) tuna, drained
- 2 tablespoons Greek yogurt
- 1 tablespoon chopped red onion
- 1/4 cup diced cucumber
- 1/4 cup diced red bell pepper

- Lettuce leaves for wrapping

Instructions:

1. In a bowl, mix together tuna, Greek yogurt, red onion, cucumber, and red bell pepper.
2. Spoon the tuna salad mixture onto lettuce leaves.
3. Roll up the lettuce leaves to form wraps, and enjoy this light and protein-packed lunch.

Chickpea and Vegetable Stir-Fry

Ingredients:

- 1 can (15 ounces) chickpeas, drained and rinsed
- 1 cup broccoli florets
- 1 cup sliced bell peppers (any color)
- 1 cup snap peas
- 2 cloves garlic, minced
- 2 tablespoons low-sodium soy sauce
- 1 tablespoon sesame oil
- 1 teaspoon grated fresh ginger
- Sesame seeds for garnish (optional)

Instructions:

1. In a large skillet or wok, heat sesame oil over medium-high heat.
2. Add garlic and ginger, and sauté for about 30 seconds.
3. Add chickpeas, broccoli, bell peppers, and snap peas to the skillet.
4. Stir-fry for 5-7 minutes until the vegetables are tender-crisp.
5. Drizzle soy sauce over the stir-fry and toss to coat.
6. Serve hot, garnished with sesame seeds if desired.

Caprese Salad

Ingredients:

- 2 large tomatoes, sliced
- 1 cup fresh mozzarella cheese, sliced
- Fresh basil leaves
- Balsamic glaze for drizzling
- Olive oil for drizzling
- Salt and pepper to taste

Instructions:

1. Arrange tomato and mozzarella slices on a serving platter, alternating them.
2. Tuck fresh basil leaves between the tomato and cheese slices.
3. Drizzle with balsamic glaze and olive oil.
4. Season with salt and pepper.
5. Serve as a refreshing and classic Caprese salad.

Lentil and Vegetable Soup

Ingredients:

- 1 cup dried green or brown lentils, rinsed and drained
- 4 cups vegetable broth
- 1 cup diced carrots
- 1 cup diced celery
- 1 cup diced onion
- 2 cloves garlic, minced
- 1 teaspoon dried thyme
- Salt and pepper to taste

Instructions:

1. In a large pot, combine lentils, vegetable broth, carrots, celery, onion, garlic, and thyme.

2. Bring to a boil, then reduce heat to a simmer.

3. Cover and cook for 30-35 minutes, or until lentils and vegetables are tender.

4. Season with salt and pepper to taste.

5. Serve this hearty lentil and vegetable soup as a comforting lunch option.

Chicken and Vegetable Bowl

Ingredients:

- 1 boneless, skinless chicken breast, cooked and sliced
- 1 cup steamed broccoli florets
- 1/2 cup sliced bell peppers (any color)
- 1/2 cup cooked brown rice
- 2 tablespoons low-sodium teriyaki sauce
- Sesame seeds for garnish (optional)

Instructions:

1. Arrange the cooked chicken, steamed broccoli, sliced bell peppers, and brown rice in a bowl.

2. Drizzle with low-sodium teriyaki sauce.

3. Toss to combine all the ingredients.

4. Garnish with sesame seeds if desired.

5. Enjoy this balanced and flavorful chicken and vegetable bowl.

Egg Salad Lettuce Wraps

Ingredients:

- 4 hard-boiled eggs, chopped
- 2 tablespoons Greek yogurt
- 1 teaspoon Dijon mustard
- 1/4 cup diced celery
- 1/4 cup diced red onion
- Lettuce leaves for wrapping
- Salt and pepper to taste

Instructions:

1. In a bowl, combine chopped hard-boiled eggs, Greek yogurt, Dijon mustard, diced celery, and diced red onion.

2. Mix until well combined.

3. Season with salt and pepper to taste.

4. Spoon the egg salad mixture onto lettuce leaves.

5. Wrap them up, and you have a low oxalate alternative to traditional egg salad sandwiches.

Cauliflower Rice Stir-Fry

Ingredients:

- 2 cups cauliflower rice
- 1 cup mixed stir-fry vegetables (e.g., broccoli, bell peppers, snap peas)
- 1/2 cup diced tofu or chicken (optional)
- 2 tablespoons low-sodium soy sauce
- 1 tablespoon sesame oil
- 1 clove garlic, minced
- 1 teaspoon grated fresh ginger
- Sesame seeds for garnish (optional)

Instructions:

1. In a large skillet, heat sesame oil over medium-high heat.
2. Add garlic and ginger, and sauté for about 30 seconds.
3. Add cauliflower rice, stir-fry vegetables, and tofu or chicken if using.
4. Stir-fry for 5-7 minutes until the cauliflower rice is tender.
5. Drizzle with low-sodium soy sauce and toss to combine.
6. Garnish with sesame seeds if desired.
7. Serve this delicious cauliflower rice stir-fry as a satisfying lunch.

Greek Salad

Ingredients:

- 2 cups chopped romaine lettuce
- 1/2 cup diced cucumber
- 1/2 cup diced tomatoes
- 1/4 cup sliced Kalamata olives
- 1/4 cup crumbled feta cheese

- Red onion slices (optional)
- Greek dressing

Instructions:

1. In a bowl, combine romaine lettuce, cucumber, tomatoes, Kalamata olives, and feta cheese.
2. Add red onion slices if desired.
3. Drizzle with your favorite Greek dressing.
4. Toss gently to coat and enjoy the fresh and tangy flavors of this Greek salad.

Zucchini Noodles with Pesto

Ingredients:

- 2 medium zucchinis, spiralized into noodles
- 1/4 cup pesto sauce (store-bought or homemade)
- Cherry tomatoes for garnish (optional)
- Grated Parmesan cheese for garnish (optional)

Instructions:

1. Spiralize the zucchinis into noodles using a spiralizer.

2. In a large bowl, toss the zucchini noodles with pesto sauce until well coated.

3. Garnish with cherry tomatoes and grated Parmesan cheese if desired.

4. Serve this light and flavorful dish as a low oxalate lunch option.

Turkey and Vegetable Soup

Ingredients:

- 1 cup cooked turkey, diced
- 2 cups mixed vegetables (carrots, celery, peas)
- 4 cups low-sodium chicken broth
- 1/2 cup diced onion
- 1 clove garlic, minced
- 1 teaspoon dried thyme
- Salt and pepper to taste

Instructions:

1. In a large pot, combine diced turkey, mixed vegetables, chicken broth, diced onion, minced garlic, and dried thyme.

2. Bring to a boil, then reduce heat and simmer for 15-20 minutes until vegetables are tender.

3. Season with salt and pepper to taste.

4. Enjoy this comforting and hearty turkey and vegetable soup.

Cucumber and Tomato Salad

Ingredients:

- 2 cups diced cucumbers
- 1 cup cherry tomatoes, halved
- 1/4 cup diced red onion
- 2 tablespoons fresh dill, chopped
- 2 tablespoons olive oil
- 1 tablespoon red wine vinegar
- Salt and pepper to taste

Instructions:

1. In a bowl, combine diced cucumbers, cherry tomatoes, diced red onion, and chopped fresh dill.

2. In a separate small bowl, whisk together olive oil, red wine vinegar, salt, and pepper.

3. Drizzle the dressing over the salad and toss to coat.

4.   Serve this crisp and refreshing cucumber and tomato salad.

Shrimp and Avocado Salad

Ingredients:

- 8-10 cooked and peeled shrimp
- 1 avocado, diced
- 1 cup mixed greens (e.g., spinach, arugula)
- 1/4 cup diced red bell pepper
- 1/4 cup diced cucumber
- Lemon vinaigrette dressing

Instructions:

1. In a bowl, combine cooked shrimp, diced avocado, mixed greens, diced red bell pepper, and diced cucumber.
2. Drizzle with lemon vinaigrette dressing.
3. Toss gently to combine.
4. Enjoy a light and protein-packed shrimp and avocado salad.

Broccoli and Cheddar Stuffed Chicken

Ingredients:

- 2 boneless, skinless chicken breasts
- 1 cup steamed broccoli florets, chopped
- 1/2 cup shredded cheddar cheese
- 1/4 cup diced red bell pepper
- 1/4 cup diced onion
- 1 clove garlic, minced
- Salt and pepper to taste

Instructions:

1. Preheat your oven to 375°F (190°C).
2. Slice a pocket into each chicken breast without cutting all the way through.
3. In a bowl, combine steamed broccoli, shredded cheddar cheese, diced red bell pepper, diced onion, minced garlic, salt, and pepper.
4. Stuff each chicken breast with the broccoli and cheese mixture.
5. Place the stuffed chicken breasts in a baking dish.

6. Bake for 25-30 minutes or until the chicken is cooked through.

7. Serve the broccoli and cheddar stuffed chicken as a hearty and flavorful lunch option.

Spinach and Mushroom Quiche

Ingredients:

- 1 pie crust (store-bought or homemade)
- 2 cups fresh spinach, chopped
- 1 cup sliced mushrooms
- 1/2 cup shredded Swiss cheese
- 4 large eggs
- 1 cup milk
- Salt and pepper to taste

Instructions:

1. Preheat your oven to 375°F (190°C).

2. Line a pie dish with the pie crust.

3. In a skillet, sauté chopped spinach and sliced mushrooms until wilted and tender.

4. Spread the spinach and mushroom mixture evenly over the pie crust.

5. Sprinkle shredded Swiss cheese on top.

6. In a bowl, whisk together eggs, milk, salt, and pepper.

7. Pour the egg mixture over the spinach, mushrooms, and cheese.

8. Bake for 35-40 minutes or until the quiche is set and lightly golden.

9. Let it cool slightly before slicing and serving this delicious spinach and mushroom quiche.

Quinoa and Vegetable Bowl

Ingredients:

- 1 cup cooked quinoa
- 1 cup mixed roasted vegetables (e.g., bell peppers, zucchini, carrots)
- 1/4 cup crumbled feta cheese
- Kalamata olives for garnish (optional)
- Greek dressing

Instructions:

1. In a bowl, combine cooked quinoa and mixed roasted vegetables.

2. Sprinkle crumbled feta cheese over the mixture.

3. Garnish with Kalamata olives if desired.

4. Drizzle with your favorite Greek dressing.

5. Toss gently to combine.

6. Enjoy this wholesome quinoa and vegetable bowl.

Chapter 4: Dinner Recipes

In this chapter, we delve into a tantalizing array of dinner recipes that are not only delicious but also adhere to a low oxalate diet. These dishes are thoughtfully crafted to provide you with a variety of flavors and ingredients to keep your dinners exciting and satisfying.

Grilled Lemon Herb Chicken

Ingredients:

- 4 boneless, skinless chicken breasts
- 2 lemons (juice and zest)
- 2 tablespoons olive oil
- 2 cloves garlic, minced
- 1 tablespoon fresh rosemary, chopped
- 1 tablespoon fresh thyme leaves
- Salt and pepper to taste

Instructions:

1. In a bowl, combine lemon juice, lemon zest, olive oil, garlic, rosemary, thyme, salt, and pepper.

2. Marinate chicken breasts in the mixture for at least 30 minutes.

3. Preheat the grill to medium-high heat.

4. Grill the chicken for 6-7 minutes per side, or until cooked through.

5. Serve with your favorite low oxalate side dishes.

Baked Salmon with Dill

Ingredients:

- 4 salmon fillets
- 2 tablespoons fresh dill, chopped
- 2 cloves garlic, minced
- 2 tablespoons olive oil
- Salt and pepper to taste
- Lemon wedges for garnish

Instructions:

1. Preheat your oven to 375°F (190°C).

2. Place salmon fillets on a baking sheet.

3. In a bowl, mix together dill, garlic, olive oil, salt, and pepper.

4. Drizzle the mixture over the salmon.

5. Bake for 15-20 minutes or until the salmon flakes easily.

6. Garnish with lemon wedges before serving.

Stir-Fried Tofu with Broccoli

Ingredients:

- 1 block of firm tofu, cubed
- 2 cups broccoli florets
- 2 tablespoons sesame oil
- 2 cloves garlic, minced
- 2 tablespoons low sodium soy sauce
- 1 tablespoon rice vinegar
- 1 teaspoon ginger, grated
- Red pepper flakes (optional)
- Sesame seeds for garnish

Instructions:

1. Heat sesame oil in a large pan or wok over medium-high heat.

2. Add cubed tofu and stir-fry until golden brown.

3. Remove tofu from the pan and set aside.

4. In the same pan, add garlic and ginger, and sauté for a minute.

5. Add broccoli and stir-fry for 3-4 minutes.

6. Return tofu to the pan, and drizzle with soy sauce and rice vinegar.

7. Toss to combine and cook for an additional 2 minutes.

8. Garnish with red pepper flakes and sesame seeds before serving.

Lemon Garlic Shrimp

Ingredients:

- 1 pound large shrimp, peeled and deveined
- 3 tablespoons olive oil
- 3 cloves garlic, minced
- Zest and juice of 1 lemon
- 2 tablespoons fresh parsley, chopped
- Salt and pepper to taste

Instructions:

1. In a bowl, combine shrimp, olive oil, garlic, lemon zest, lemon juice, parsley, salt, and pepper.

2. Let the shrimp marinate for 15-20 minutes.

3. Heat a skillet over medium-high heat.

4. Add the shrimp and cook for 2-3 minutes per side until they turn pink and opaque.

5. Serve hot with your favorite low oxalate side dishes.

Roasted Vegetable Medley

Ingredients:

- 2 cups mixed low oxalate vegetables (e.g., bell peppers, zucchini, carrots)
- 2 tablespoons olive oil
- 1 teaspoon dried Italian herbs
- Salt and pepper to taste

Instructions:

1. Preheat your oven to 400°F (200°C).

2. Cut the vegetables into bite-sized pieces.

3. Toss the vegetables with olive oil, Italian herbs, salt, and pepper.

4. Spread them on a baking sheet in a single layer.

5. Roast for 20-25 minutes or until they are tender and slightly caramelized.

6. Serve as a side dish or over cooked quinoa or rice.

Turkey Meatballs in Tomato Sauce

Ingredients:

- 1 pound ground turkey
- 1/2 cup breadcrumbs (use a low oxalate option)
- 1/4 cup grated Parmesan cheese
- 1 egg
- 2 cloves garlic, minced
- 1 teaspoon dried oregano
- Salt and pepper to taste
- 1 can low oxalate tomato sauce

Instructions:

1. Preheat your oven to 375°F (190°C).
2. In a bowl, combine ground turkey, breadcrumbs, Parmesan cheese, egg, garlic, oregano, salt, and pepper.
3. Form the mixture into meatballs and place them in a baking dish.
4. Pour tomato sauce over the meatballs.

5. Bake for 25-30 minutes or until the meatballs are cooked through.

6. Serve over low oxalate pasta or with a side of vegetables.

Baked Cod with Herbs

Ingredients:

- 4 cod fillets
- 2 tablespoons olive oil
- 2 cloves garlic, minced
- 1 tablespoon fresh dill, chopped
- 1 tablespoon fresh parsley, chopped
- Zest and juice of 1 lemon
- Salt and pepper to taste

Instructions:

1. Preheat your oven to 375°F (190°C).

2. Place cod fillets in a baking dish.

3. In a bowl, mix together olive oil, garlic, dill, parsley, lemon zest, lemon juice, salt, and pepper.

4. Drizzle the mixture over the cod.

5. Bake for 15-20 minutes or until the cod flakes easily with a fork.

6. Serve with a side of steamed low oxalate vegetables.

Beef and Broccoli Stir-Fry

Ingredients:

- 1 pound lean beef, thinly sliced
- 2 cups broccoli florets
- 2 tablespoons low sodium soy sauce
- 1 tablespoon oyster sauce
- 2 cloves garlic, minced
- 1 teaspoon ginger, grated
- 1 tablespoon vegetable oil
- Sesame seeds for garnish

Instructions:

1. In a bowl, combine sliced beef, soy sauce, oyster sauce, garlic, and ginger.

2. Heat vegetable oil in a large skillet or wok over high heat.

3. Add the marinated beef and stir-fry for 2-3 minutes until browned.

4. Add broccoli and continue to stir-fry for an additional 3-4 minutes until tender.

5. Garnish with sesame seeds before serving.

Spaghetti Squash with Pesto

Ingredients:

- 1 spaghetti squash
- 2 tablespoons olive oil
- 1/2 cup low oxalate pesto sauce (store-bought or homemade)
- Grated Parmesan cheese for garnish
- Fresh basil leaves for garnish (optional)

Instructions:

1. Preheat your oven to 375°F (190°C).

2. Cut the spaghetti squash in half lengthwise and remove the seeds.

3. Drizzle olive oil over the cut sides of the squash and season with salt and pepper.

4. Place the squash halves cut-side down on a baking sheet and roast for 40-45 minutes, or until the flesh is tender.

5. Use a fork to scrape the squash into spaghetti-like strands.

6. Toss the spaghetti squash with pesto sauce until well coated.

7. Garnish with grated Parmesan cheese and fresh basil leaves.

Pork Tenderloin with Apple Glaze

Ingredients:

- 2 pork tenderloins
- 2 apples, peeled, cored, and sliced
- 1/4 cup apple juice
- 2 tablespoons brown sugar
- 2 tablespoons Dijon mustard
- 2 cloves garlic, minced
- Salt and pepper to taste

Instructions:

1. Preheat your oven to 375°F (190°C).

2. Season pork tenderloins with salt and pepper.

3. In a large ovenproof skillet, sear the pork on all sides until browned.

4. In a separate bowl, combine apple juice, brown sugar, Dijon mustard, and garlic.

5. Pour the mixture over the pork.

6. Add apple slices to the skillet.

7. Transfer the skillet to the oven and roast for 20-25 minutes, or until the pork reaches an internal temperature of 145°F (63°C).

8. Let the pork rest for a few minutes before slicing.

9. Serve with the apple glaze and roasted apples.

Baked Eggplant Parmesan

Ingredients:

- 2 large eggplants, sliced into rounds
- 1 cup low oxalate marinara sauce
- 1 cup shredded mozzarella cheese
- 1/2 cup grated Parmesan cheese
- 1/4 cup fresh basil leaves, chopped
- 2 tablespoons olive oil
- Salt and pepper to taste

Instructions:

1. Preheat your oven to 375°F (190°C).

2. Arrange eggplant slices on a baking sheet and brush with olive oil.

3. Season with salt and pepper.

4. Bake for 15-20 minutes until the eggplant is tender.

5. In a baking dish, layer marinara sauce, eggplant slices, mozzarella cheese, Parmesan cheese, and basil.

6. Repeat the layers.

7. Bake for 20-25 minutes, or until the cheese is bubbly and golden.

8. Let it cool slightly before serving.

Chicken and Asparagus Stir-Fry

Ingredients:

- 2 boneless, skinless chicken breasts, cut into thin strips
- 1 bunch fresh asparagus, trimmed and cut into bite-sized pieces
- 2 cloves garlic, minced
- 1 tablespoon low sodium soy sauce
- 1 tablespoon oyster sauce
- 1 tablespoon vegetable oil

- Sesame seeds for garnish (optional)

Instructions:

1. In a bowl, mix chicken strips with soy sauce and oyster sauce.
2. Heat vegetable oil in a large skillet or wok over medium-high heat.
3. Add minced garlic and sauté for a minute.
4. Add chicken and stir-fry until cooked through, about 5-6 minutes.
5. Add asparagus and continue to stir-fry for another 3-4 minutes until tender.
6. Garnish with sesame seeds if desired before serving.

Grilled Portobello Mushrooms

Ingredients:

- 4 large Portobello mushrooms, stems removed
- 2 tablespoons balsamic vinegar
- 2 cloves garlic, minced
- 2 tablespoons olive oil
- Salt and pepper to taste
- Fresh parsley for garnish

Instructions:

1. Preheat your grill to medium-high heat.

2. In a bowl, whisk together balsamic vinegar, garlic, olive oil, salt, and pepper.

3. Brush the mixture over the mushroom caps.

4. Grill the mushrooms for 4-5 minutes per side until they are tender.

5. Garnish with fresh parsley before serving.

Stuffed Bell Peppers

Ingredients:

- 4 bell peppers, any color
- 1 pound lean ground beef
- 1 cup cooked rice (use a low oxalate variety)
- 1 can low oxalate tomato sauce
- 1 onion, finely chopped
- 2 cloves garlic, minced
- 1 teaspoon dried Italian herbs
- Salt and pepper to taste
- Shredded mozzarella cheese for topping

Instructions:

1. Preheat your oven to 375°F (190°C).

2. Cut the tops off the bell peppers and remove the seeds and membranes.

3. In a skillet, brown ground beef with onion and garlic until cooked through.

4. Stir in cooked rice, tomato sauce, Italian herbs, salt, and pepper.

5. Fill each bell pepper with the beef and rice mixture.

6. Place the peppers in a baking dish and top with mozzarella cheese.

7. Bake for 25-30 minutes or until the peppers are tender and the cheese is melted and bubbly.

Balsamic Glazed Brussels Sprouts

Ingredients:

- 1 pound Brussels sprouts, trimmed and halved
- 2 tablespoons olive oil
- 2 tablespoons balsamic vinegar
- 2 cloves garlic, minced
- Salt and pepper to taste

Instructions:

1. Preheat your oven to 400°F (200°C).

2. Toss Brussels sprouts with olive oil, balsamic vinegar, garlic, salt, and pepper.

3. Spread them on a baking sheet in a single layer.

4. Roast for 20-25 minutes, stirring halfway through, until they are caramelized and tender.

5. Serve hot as a side dish.

Cilantro Lime Cauliflower Rice

Ingredients:

- 1 head cauliflower, riced
- Juice and zest of 2 limes
- 1/4 cup fresh cilantro, chopped
- 2 cloves garlic, minced
- 2 tablespoons olive oil
- Salt and pepper to taste

Instructions:

1. Heat olive oil in a large skillet over medium heat.

2. Add minced garlic and sauté for a minute.

3. Add cauliflower rice and cook for 5-7 minutes, stirring occasionally, until tender.

4. Stir in lime juice, lime zest, cilantro, salt, and pepper.

5. Cook for an additional 2 minutes before serving.

Lemon Butter Tilapia

Ingredients:

- 4 tilapia fillets
- 2 tablespoons unsalted butter
- Juice and zest of 1 lemon
- 2 cloves garlic, minced
- 1 tablespoon fresh parsley, chopped
- Salt and pepper to taste

Instructions:

1. In a skillet, melt butter over medium heat.

2. Add minced garlic and sauté for a minute.

3. Place tilapia fillets in the skillet.

4. Season with salt, pepper, and lemon zest.

5. Cook for 3-4 minutes per side or until the fish flakes easily.

6. Drizzle with lemon juice and garnish with fresh parsley before serving.

Ratatouille

Ingredients:

- 2 zucchinis, sliced
- 1 eggplant, sliced
- 2 tomatoes, sliced
- 1 bell pepper, sliced
- 1 onion, sliced
- 2 cloves garlic, minced
- 2 tablespoons olive oil
- 1 teaspoon dried thyme
- Salt and pepper to taste
- Fresh basil leaves for garnish

Instructions:

1. Preheat your oven to 375°F (190°C).
2. In a baking dish, arrange alternating slices of zucchini, eggplant, tomato, bell pepper, and onion.
3. Sprinkle minced garlic over the top.
4. Drizzle olive oil and sprinkle thyme, salt, and pepper.

5. Cover with foil and bake for 45-50 minutes.

6. Remove the foil and bake for an additional 15-20 minutes until vegetables are tender.

7. Garnish with fresh basil leaves before serving.

Chapter 5: Snacks and Appetizers

In this chapter, we dive into a delightful array of snacks and appetizers that not only satisfy your cravings but also align with a low oxalate diet. These recipes are perfect for those in-between moments or for impressing your guests with wholesome nibbles.

Guacamole with Veggie Sticks

Ingredients:

- 2 ripe avocados
- 1 small red onion, finely diced
- 2 cloves garlic, minced
- 1-2 tomatoes, diced
- 1 lime, juiced
- Salt and pepper to taste
- Assorted veggie sticks (carrots, celery, cucumber) for dipping

Instructions:

1. Cut the avocados in half, remove the pits, and scoop the flesh into a bowl.
2. Mash the avocados with a fork, leaving some chunks for texture.
3. Add the diced onion, minced garlic, diced tomatoes, and lime juice to the bowl. Mix well.
4. Season with salt and pepper to taste.
5. Serve with a colorful assortment of veggie sticks for dipping.

Hummus and Carrot Slices

Ingredients:

- 1 can (15 oz) chickpeas, drained and rinsed
- 1/4 cup tahini
- 2 cloves garlic, minced
- 2 tablespoons lemon juice
- 2 tablespoons olive oil
- 1/2 teaspoon ground cumin
- Salt and paprika to taste
- Carrot slices for dipping

Instructions:

1. In a food processor, combine chickpeas, tahini, minced garlic, lemon juice, olive oil, cumin, salt, and paprika.
2. Blend until smooth, adding a splash of water if needed to reach your desired consistency.
3. Transfer to a serving dish and drizzle with a bit of olive oil.
4. Serve with fresh carrot slices for a crunchy and creamy snack.

Greek Yogurt with Berries

Ingredients:

- 1 cup Greek yogurt
- 1/2 cup mixed berries (strawberries, blueberries, raspberries)
- 1 tablespoon honey (optional)

Instructions:

1. Spoon the Greek yogurt into a bowl or serving glass.
2. Top with a generous handful of mixed berries.

3. Drizzle with honey if you prefer a touch of sweetness.

4. Enjoy this nutritious and satisfying yogurt and berry combination.

Cucumber Slices with Tzatziki

Ingredients:

- 1 cucumber
- 1 cup Greek yogurt
- 1 clove garlic, minced
- 1 tablespoon fresh dill, chopped
- 1/2 lemon, juiced
- Salt and pepper to taste

Instructions:

1. Peel the cucumber and slice it thinly.

2. In a bowl, mix Greek yogurt, minced garlic, fresh dill, lemon juice, salt, and pepper.

3. Serve the cucumber slices with a side of homemade tzatziki sauce for a refreshing and tangy snack.

Almonds and Dried Cranberries

Ingredients:

- 1 cup almonds
- 1/2 cup dried cranberries

Instructions:

1. Combine the almonds and dried cranberries in a bowl.
2. Mix well to create a satisfying blend of nutty and fruity flavors.
3. This simple combination makes for a healthy and delicious snack.

Roasted Red Pepper Dip

Ingredients:

- 2 red bell peppers
- 1/4 cup Greek yogurt
- 2 cloves garlic, minced
- 1 tablespoon olive oil
- Salt and pepper to taste
- Fresh parsley for garnish

- Assorted veggie sticks or pita bread for dipping

Instructions:

1. Roast the red bell peppers over an open flame or under a broiler until charred.
2. Place the roasted peppers in a bowl, cover with plastic wrap, and let them steam for about 10 minutes.
3. Peel off the charred skin, remove the seeds, and chop the peppers.
4. In a blender or food processor, combine the roasted peppers, Greek yogurt, minced garlic, olive oil, salt, and pepper.
5. Blend until smooth.
6. Garnish with fresh parsley and serve with veggie sticks or pita bread.

Deviled Eggs

Ingredients:

- 6 hard-boiled eggs, peeled
- 2 tablespoons Greek yogurt
- 1 teaspoon Dijon mustard

- Salt and paprika to taste
- Fresh chives for garnish

Instructions:

1. Cut the hard-boiled eggs in half lengthwise.
2. Remove the yolks and place them in a bowl.
3. Mash the yolks with Greek yogurt, Dijon mustard, salt, and paprika until creamy.
4. Spoon the yolk mixture back into the egg whites.
5. Garnish with fresh chives.
6. These classic deviled eggs are sure to please any crowd.

Cottage Cheese with Pineapple

Ingredients:

- 1 cup low-fat cottage cheese
- 1/2 cup fresh pineapple chunks

Instructions:

1. In a serving bowl, spoon the low-fat cottage cheese.
2. Top it with fresh pineapple chunks.

3. This combination of creamy cottage cheese and sweet pineapple is a delightful, protein-rich snack.

Stuffed Mushrooms

Ingredients:

- 12 large mushroom caps
- 1/2 cup cream cheese
- 2 cloves garlic, minced
- 2 tablespoons grated Parmesan cheese
- Fresh parsley for garnish

Instructions:

1. Preheat your oven to 350°F (175°C).
2. Clean the mushroom caps and remove the stems.
3. In a bowl, mix cream cheese, minced garlic, and grated Parmesan cheese.
4. Stuff each mushroom cap with the cream cheese mixture.
5. Place the stuffed mushrooms on a baking sheet and bake for 15-20 minutes or until they are tender.
6. Garnish with fresh parsley before serving.

Edamame with Sea Salt

Ingredients:

- 1 cup edamame (young soybeans), steamed
- Sea salt to taste

Instructions:

1. Steam the edamame according to the package instructions.
2. Sprinkle with sea salt to taste.
3. Edamame pods are a delightful and nutritious snack, perfect for satisfying your cravings.

Avocado Salsa

Ingredients:

- 2 ripe avocados, diced
- 1 tomato, diced
- 1/2 red onion, finely chopped
- 1/4 cup fresh cilantro, chopped
- 1 lime, juiced
- Salt and pepper to taste

Instructions:

1. In a bowl, combine diced avocados, diced tomato, chopped red onion, fresh cilantro, lime juice, salt, and pepper.

2. Gently toss to mix all the ingredients.

3. Serve this refreshing avocado salsa with your favorite whole-grain crackers or tortilla chips.

Baked Sweet Potato Fries

Ingredients:

- 2 large sweet potatoes, cut into fries
- 2 tablespoons olive oil
- 1/2 teaspoon paprika
- Salt and pepper to taste

Instructions:

1. Preheat your oven to 425°F (220°C).

2. Toss sweet potato fries with olive oil, paprika, salt, and pepper.

3. Spread them in a single layer on a baking sheet.

4. Bake for 20-25 minutes or until the fries are crispy and golden brown.

5. Serve these homemade sweet potato fries as a healthier alternative to traditional fries.

Caprese Skewers

Ingredients:

- Cherry tomatoes
- Fresh mozzarella balls
- Fresh basil leaves
- Balsamic glaze
- Skewers or toothpicks

Instructions:

1. Thread a cherry tomato, a fresh mozzarella ball, and a fresh basil leaf onto a skewer or toothpick.
2. Arrange the skewers on a plate.
3. Drizzle with balsamic glaze for a burst of flavor.
4. These Caprese skewers are a delightful and elegant appetizer.

Mixed Nuts

Ingredients:

- A mixture of your favorite nuts (almonds, cashews, walnuts, etc.)

Instructions:

1. Simply combine your preferred nuts in a bowl or create your own custom mix.
2. Enjoy the natural goodness and crunch of mixed nuts as a satisfying snack.

Cucumber and Cream Cheese Roll-Ups

Ingredients:

- 1 cucumber
- Cream cheese
- Smoked salmon (optional)
- Fresh dill (optional)

Instructions:

1. Slice the cucumber thinly lengthwise.

2. Spread cream cheese on each cucumber slice.

3. Add a thin slice of smoked salmon, if desired.

4. Roll up the cucumber slices.

5. Garnish with fresh dill, if you like.

6. These roll-ups are both refreshing and indulgent.

Sliced Bell Peppers with Ranch Dressing

Ingredients:

- Bell peppers, various colors, sliced
- Ranch dressing for dipping

Instructions:

1. Slice bell peppers into strips.

2. Serve with a side of creamy ranch dressing for dipping.

3. Enjoy the crispness of bell peppers with the rich flavor of ranch.

Zucchini Chips

Ingredients:

- 2 medium zucchinis, thinly sliced
- Olive oil spray
- Salt and garlic powder to taste

Instructions:

1. Preheat your oven to 225°F (110°C).
2. Lay zucchini slices on a baking sheet and lightly spray with olive oil.
3. Sprinkle with salt and garlic powder.
4. Bake for 2-3 hours until they become crispy.
5. These zucchini chips are a nutritious alternative to traditional potato chips.

Kale Chips

Ingredients:

- Fresh kale leaves, stems removed and torn into pieces
- Olive oil spray

- Seasonings of your choice (salt, paprika, nutritional yeast, etc.)

Instructions:

1. Preheat your oven to 275°F (135°C).
2. Place kale pieces on a baking sheet and spray with olive oil.
3. Sprinkle with your preferred seasonings.
4. Bake for 15-20 minutes until kale becomes crispy.
5. Enjoy these guilt-free kale chips for a crunchy snack.

Chapter 6: Desserts

In this chapter, we've curated a collection of sweet treats that are not only scrumptious but also mindful of your dietary needs. From fruity sorbets to indulgent chocolate creations, there's something here to satisfy every sweet tooth while keeping oxalate levels in check.

Low Oxalate Berry Sorbet

Ingredients:

- 2 cups mixed berries (strawberries, blueberries, raspberries)
- 1/4 cup honey or maple syrup
- 1 tablespoon lemon juice

Instructions:

1. Blend the berries until smooth.
2. Add honey or maple syrup and lemon juice, then blend again.
3. Pour the mixture into a freezer-safe container and freeze for at least 4 hours. Scoop and enjoy!

Chocolate Avocado Mousse

Ingredients:

- 2 ripe avocados
- 1/4 cup cocoa powder
- 1/4 cup honey or agave nectar
- 1 teaspoon vanilla extract

Instructions:

1. Blend avocados, cocoa powder, honey, and vanilla extract until creamy.
2. Chill in the fridge for 30 minutes before serving. Top with berries or nuts if desired.

Almond Flour Brownies

Ingredients:

- 2 cups almond flour
- 1/2 cup cocoa powder
- 1/2 cup honey
- 2 eggs
- 1/4 cup coconut oil
- 1 teaspoon vanilla extract

- 1/2 teaspoon baking soda
- Pinch of salt

Instructions:

1. Preheat your oven to 350°F (175°C).
2. In a bowl, mix almond flour, cocoa powder, baking soda, and salt.
3. In another bowl, whisk honey, eggs, melted coconut oil, and vanilla extract.
4. Combine wet and dry ingredients, then pour into a greased baking pan.
5. Bake for 25-30 minutes. Allow to cool before cutting into squares.

Baked Apple with Cinnamon

Ingredients:

- 4 apples, cored and halved
- 1 teaspoon cinnamon
- 2 tablespoons honey

Instructions:

1. Preheat your oven to 350°F (175°C).

2. Place apple halves in a baking dish, sprinkle with cinnamon, and drizzle honey over them.

3. Bake for 20-25 minutes until apples are tender. Serve warm.

Lemon Poppy Seed Cake

Ingredients:

- 2 cups almond flour
- 1/4 cup poppy seeds
- 1/4 cup honey
- 1/4 cup lemon juice
- Zest of 1 lemon
- 3 eggs
- 1 teaspoon baking powder
- 1/2 teaspoon vanilla extract
- Pinch of salt

Instructions:

1. Preheat your oven to 350°F (175°C).

2. In a bowl, mix almond flour, poppy seeds, baking powder, and a pinch of salt.

3. In another bowl, whisk together honey, lemon juice, lemon zest, eggs, and vanilla extract.

4. Combine wet and dry ingredients, then pour the batter into a greased cake pan.

5. Bake for 30-35 minutes or until a toothpick comes out clean. Let it cool before slicing.

Coconut Milk Ice Cream

Ingredients:

- 2 cans of full-fat coconut milk
- 1/2 cup honey or agave nectar
- 1 teaspoon vanilla extract

Instructions:

1. Mix coconut milk, honey, and vanilla extract in a blender.

2. Pour the mixture into an ice cream maker and churn according to the manufacturer's instructions.

3. Freeze for a few hours to firm it up, then scoop and serve.

Banana Nut Muffins

Ingredients:

- 2 ripe bananas, mashed
- 1/4 cup almond flour
- 1/4 cup coconut flour
- 1/4 cup honey
- 2 eggs
- 1/4 cup chopped nuts (e.g., walnuts or pecans)
- 1 teaspoon baking powder
- 1/2 teaspoon cinnamon
- Pinch of salt

Instructions:

1. Preheat your oven to 350°F (175°C).
2. In a bowl, combine mashed bananas, almond flour, coconut flour, honey, eggs, chopped nuts, baking powder, cinnamon, and a pinch of salt.
3. Spoon the batter into muffin cups and bake for 20-25 minutes until golden brown.

Greek Yogurt with Honey and Nuts

Ingredients:

- 1 cup Greek yogurt
- 2 tablespoons honey
- 2 tablespoons chopped nuts (e.g., almonds or walnuts)

Instructions:

1. In a bowl, spoon the Greek yogurt.
2. Drizzle honey over the yogurt.
3. Sprinkle chopped nuts on top.
4. Stir gently to combine. Enjoy as a simple and healthy dessert.

Chia Seed Chocolate Pudding

Ingredients:

- 1/4 cup chia seeds
- 1 cup almond milk
- 2 tablespoons cocoa powder
- 2 tablespoons honey
- 1/2 teaspoon vanilla extract

- Pinch of salt

Instructions:

1. In a bowl, whisk together chia seeds, almond milk, cocoa powder, honey, vanilla extract, and a pinch of salt.
2. Refrigerate for at least 2 hours or until the mixture thickens to a pudding-like consistency.
3. Serve chilled with your choice of toppings like berries or shredded coconut.

Strawberry Shortcake

Ingredients:

- 2 cups almond flour
- 1/4 cup honey
- 2 eggs
- 1/4 cup coconut oil
- 1/2 teaspoon vanilla extract
- 1/2 teaspoon baking soda
- Pinch of salt
- Fresh strawberries

Instructions:

1. Preheat your oven to 350°F (175°C).

2. Mix almond flour, honey, eggs, melted coconut oil, vanilla extract, baking soda, and a pinch of salt in a bowl.

3. Drop spoonfuls of the batter onto a baking sheet and flatten slightly.

4. Bake for 10-12 minutes until golden.

5. Once cooled, slice the shortcakes in half, add fresh strawberries, and a dollop of Greek yogurt or whipped cream if desired.

Pumpkin Pie Bites

Ingredients:

- 1 cup canned pumpkin puree
- 1/4 cup almond flour
- 1/4 cup honey
- 1 egg
- 1 teaspoon pumpkin pie spice
- 1/2 teaspoon vanilla extract
- Pinch of salt

Instructions:

1. Preheat your oven to 350°F (175°C).
2. In a bowl, mix pumpkin puree, almond flour, honey, egg, pumpkin pie spice, vanilla extract, and a pinch of salt.
3. Spoon the mixture into mini muffin cups.
4. Bake for 18-20 minutes or until set. Let them cool before removing from the pan.

Mango Sorbet

Ingredients:

- 2 ripe mangoes, peeled and diced
- 1/4 cup honey or agave nectar
- Juice of 1 lime

Instructions:

1. Blend mangoes, honey, and lime juice until smooth.
2. Pour the mixture into a freezer-safe container and freeze for at least 4 hours. Scoop and enjoy!

Raspberry Cheesecake Bars

Ingredients:

- 1 cup almond flour
- 1/4 cup honey
- 8 oz cream cheese, softened
- 1 egg
- 1 teaspoon vanilla extract
- 1/2 cup fresh raspberries

Instructions:

1. Preheat your oven to 350°F (175°C).
2. In a bowl, mix almond flour and honey to form the crust.
3. Press the crust into a greased baking dish.
4. In another bowl, beat cream cheese, egg, and vanilla extract until smooth.
5. Pour the cream cheese mixture over the crust.
6. Drop fresh raspberries on top.
7. Bake for 25-30 minutes or until set. Let it cool before cutting into bars.

Almond and Date Energy Balls

Ingredients:

- 1 cup almonds
- 1 cup pitted dates
- 1/4 cup unsweetened shredded coconut
- 1/4 cup cocoa powder
- 1/2 teaspoon vanilla extract

Instructions:

1. Combine almonds, dates, shredded coconut, cocoa powder, and vanilla extract in a food processor.
2. Pulse until the mixture comes together.
3. Roll the mixture into small energy balls.

Carrot Cake Bites

Ingredients:

- 1 cup almond flour
- 1/4 cup honey
- 1 cup shredded carrots
- 1/4 cup chopped nuts (e.g., walnuts or pecans)
- 1/2 teaspoon cinnamon

- Pinch of salt

Instructions:

1. In a bowl, mix almond flour, honey, shredded carrots, chopped nuts, cinnamon, and a pinch of salt.
2. Roll the mixture into bite-sized balls.

Blueberry Crumble

Ingredients:

- 2 cups blueberries
- 1/2 cup almond flour
- 1/4 cup honey
- 1/4 cup rolled oats
- 1/4 cup coconut oil
- 1/2 teaspoon cinnamon
- Pinch of salt

Instructions:

1. Preheat your oven to 350°F (175°C).
2. In a bowl, toss blueberries with a drizzle of honey.

3. In another bowl, combine almond flour, rolled oats, melted coconut oil, cinnamon, and a pinch of salt to make the crumble topping.

4. Spread the blueberries in a baking dish and top with the crumble mixture.

5. Bake for 30-35 minutes or until the topping is golden and the blueberries are bubbly.

Chocolate-Dipped Strawberries

Ingredients:

- Fresh strawberries
- Dark chocolate chips (low oxalate)
- Coconut oil (for melting chocolate)

Instructions:

1. Melt dark chocolate chips with a bit of coconut oil in a microwave or double boiler.

2. Dip fresh strawberries into the melted chocolate.

3. Place them on a parchment paper-lined tray and refrigerate until the chocolate hardens.

Pecan Pie Squares

Ingredients:

- 1 cup almond flour
- 1/4 cup honey
- 2 eggs
- 1 cup chopped pecans
- 1/4 cup coconut oil
- 1/2 teaspoon vanilla extract
- Pinch of salt

Instructions:

1. Preheat your oven to 350°F (175°C).
2. In a bowl, mix almond flour, honey, eggs, chopped pecans, melted coconut oil, vanilla extract, and a pinch of salt.
3. Spread the mixture in a baking dish and bake for 25-30 minutes or until set. Let it cool before cutting into squares.

CONCLUSION

As we reach the final chapter of the "Low Oxalate Cookbook," it's time to reflect on the journey you've embarked upon. This concluding section isn't just about closing the book; it's about opening a door to a healthier lifestyle that's sustainable and satisfying.

Your Journey, Your Success

Throughout this cookbook, you've discovered a multitude of delicious low oxalate recipes to tantalize your taste buds and support your well-being. But remember, this journey is uniquely yours. It's not about perfection; it's about progress. Whether you're managing a medical condition or simply seeking a healthier lifestyle, your dedication is commendable.

Staying on a Low Oxalate Diet

Now, the question arises: "How do you maintain this low oxalate lifestyle beyond these pages?" The answer lies in creating a sustainable plan that works for you. Consider these tips:

1. Meal Planning: Continue to plan your meals ahead of time. This not only ensures you have the right ingredients but also saves you time and reduces the temptation to stray from your dietary goals.

2. Variety is Key: Explore new recipes and ingredients regularly. Keeping your meals exciting and diverse makes it easier to stick to your low oxalate diet.

3. Mindful Eating: Practice mindful eating by savoring each bite. Pay attention to your body's hunger and fullness cues. This can help prevent overeating and improve your overall relationship with food.

4. Stay Hydrated: Drinking enough water is crucial. It not only supports overall health but also helps flush excess oxalates from your system.

Tips for Long-Term Success

Achieving long-term success on a low oxalate diet goes beyond the kitchen. Here are some lifestyle tips to support your journey:

1. Stay Informed: Keep up with the latest research and developments related to oxalates and dietary recommendations. Knowledge is your ally.

2. Find Support: Share your journey with friends and family. Their support can be invaluable, and you might even inspire them to adopt healthier eating habits.

3. Celebrate Small Wins: Don't forget to celebrate your achievements, no matter how small. Each step you take toward a healthier you is worth acknowledging.

4. Balance and Moderation: Remember, balance is key. While this cookbook focuses on low oxalate recipes, occasional indulgences are okay. It's about overall dietary patterns.

5. Enjoy the Process: Embrace the joy of cooking and eating. Food should be a source of pleasure as well as nourishment.

Thank you for embarking on this culinary adventure with us. Your commitment to better health is commendable, and remember, every meal is a chance to nourish both body and soul. Cheers to your continued success on your low oxalate journey!